"When I first met Elizabeth Bayer she had the worst case of ulcerative colitis I had ever seen. I recommended immediate surgery and Elizabeth's response was, "Just so you know, I don't own this!" She obviously knew something about herself that not even I, as her doctor, could recognize.

Elizabeth's commitment to positive communication, her stubborn insistence on asking all the necessary questions, and, above all, her great humanity, created an environment which genuinely affected the normal psychology of the doctor-patient relationship.

Her wisdom, her humility and her loving kindness not only had a great bearing on Elizabeth's own survival — they altered my approach to treating her, and future patients, before and after surgery, and throughout their entire recovery period.

Elizabeth's insights could be of huge value to anyone, patient and medical professionals, alike, facing the fearful realities of cancer.

I highly recommend that attending physicians keep three copies of Elizabeth's book in their office — one to read, themselves, a second for their staff to share, and a third in their reception area, for all of their patients' benefit."

~Becky Natrajan, M.D., P.C.

Contents

Introduction

CANCER.

The word immediately evokes thoughts of suffering, fear, and drama.

It carries the negative imprint of all that our society has come to know about the disease—the stigmas, the misconceptions, and the assumptions that it's a death sentence. Sadly, little of our basic understanding of cancer is ever positive.

But what if we stopped viewing cancer as a war, as something to fight *against*?

What if a new perspective offered those with a cancer diagnosis the tools to design a gentle and beautiful journey—one that flowed *with* the current—empowering them to reclaim their life along the way?

In my moment of greatest vulnerability, I learned to embrace the journey, so I could truly heal and grow. It doesn't mean that there haven't been moments that suck—there have been, most assuredly. But I've learned about the power of will and intention, and how to carry faith deep in my heart.

Can you think of one good reason *not* to create a higher story for your life? It's about self-empowerment, and nobody can do it, except you.

It's Just a Word is about how one can choose to accept a cancer diagnosis and move through all that it brings with gratitude and love.

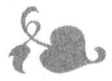

~CHAPTER ONE~

"Language-ing"

IT WAS MID-JUNE, 2005, when I received the phone call—at work, no less.

"Hi, Elizabeth, it's Becky [my gastroenterologist]. I'm shocked. Your pathology came back, and it's showing cancer. We must have caught it right when it turned."

The story you tell yourself, right from the start, is the story that will determine your outcome. It's not the story the doctors tell you or the stories you hear about other people. It's your story that matters. And it's up to you to create one that makes sense for your life, and know, that as the story changes, so do you.

So, rather than immediately download all the fearful images that would negatively imprint my energy field, I chose to "language" the news like this: "I have been diagnosed with cancer."

Take a moment and feel the difference between saying, "I *have* cancer" and "I have been *diagnosed* with cancer."

Breathe on it. You'll find that saying it the second way gives you a degree of separation and detachment that is both empowering and liberating.

This doesn't mean that you're in denial. It simply means that you don't have to carry everybody else's baggage about the word (including your own). Personally, it has allowed me to move through all of this in a much gentler way.

If you, a loved one, or someone you know has been diagnosed with cancer, it's time to reconsider the language we use to announce it. Moving toward a more positive place, we might ask: What if cancer didn't happen TO you? What if it happened FOR you?

That simple shift, from TO to FOR opens up an entirely different dialogue!

Consider the first way: Cancer happened TO you.

From the onset, language-ing it this way makes you a victim.

What are the words and feelings most commonly associated with the word, "victim?" According to the *American Heritage Dictionary of the English Language*, a "victim" is defined as "an unfortunate person who suffers from some adverse circumstance."

There are many ways to trade on the currency of being a victim, but are any of them positive or empowering? Being a victim can garner you attention, but is negative attention what you really want? Most often, people who feel sorry for you want to flee, not remain by your side. Victim-hood also requires a lot of thought and energy, all of which could be put to better use in helping you heal. There's a difference between being a victim of circumstance, and being a victim by choice, and trading on the currency of any disease is a choice.

So, what if cancer happened FOR you?

Suddenly, you're giving yourself an opportunity to learn, grow, and heal. By its nature, it brings up a myriad of other questions: What is this showing me? What are the gifts? How can this be of value to my life, or the lives of those around me?

When cancer happens FOR you, there are many possibilities:

It can be a wake-up call for how you've treated your body thus far and how you'll do so in the future. It can show you how many people in the world love you. It can teach you compassion, for yourself and for others.

It can put you in tune with the strength you never knew you possessed. It can propel you to do all the things you thought you had time for, but never did. It can help you cherish the present moment. It can assist you in offering forgiveness, and being forgiven by others. It can teach you humility and gratitude. It can help you ask better questions. It can move you toward a life with more meaning. It can raise you up to a higher level of spirituality, even if that was never part of your life. It can help you let go of the things that are not truly important to you. It can make you a better person, for yourself and the world around you.

The question is not, "Why me?" The question is, "Why NOT me?"

Starting from that place will help you be positive and bring meaning to your journey.

I was turning 40 when I was first told in 1997 that I would need to have my colon removed. At that time, there was no pathology indicating cancer. Single, and longing for a relationship, I thought, "If I'm having trouble finding a mate now, how will I ever find anyone if I'm wearing a colostomy bag? I'd been suffering from ulcerative colitis for the past fifteen years and I had to know where every public bathroom in town was located. The condition creates a spontaneous urgency to move the bowels, which absolutely will not wait for even five minutes.

In 1997, my situation was all about death. Luckily, I found amazing teachers and colleagues at The Way of the Heart who gave me the tools to do my inner, spiritual work, which put me in a position to say "yes" to whatever was going to unfold. I will always believe that my sheer willingness to do whatever was asked of me made a difference in how I ended up traveling the path — with the grace, dignity, beauty, and humor that I had set out to create. In 2005, as I began to see the divine hand in all of my struggles, it became very much about life! How glorious!

After Becky broke the news, I hung up the phone and decided right then and there that I wasn't going to own the disease. Healing begins with how you speak to yourself, and subsequently to others, and it applies to all aspects of your life. It can change everything for the better.

I said to myself, "I have been diagnosed with rectal cancer." I used that phrase to deliver the news to my family and friends.

When their first tendency was to organize a pity party (trust me-it

was) my answer to them was, "Don't feel sorry for me. It's the end of my pain and suffering."

Stopped them (dead) in their tracks. If you don't go there, they won't either. Everyone in my life was instructed that, if they needed to tell other people about my condition, the language they were to use was, "Elizabeth has been diagnosed with rectal cancer." I figured, if I'm not owning it, don't you make me own it by projecting the "she has" onto me. To a person, everyone got it, respected it, and used the specific language we all came to prefer.

For most people, CANCER is a big, bad word. In my world, it's become a word surrounded by life and beauty.

NOTE: *It's my fervent wish that doctors who deliver this news all day long will make a greater effort to assist their patients by rewording their presentations. How much gentler would it be to hear from the onset, "You have been diagnosed with _____" rather than, "You have _____"? If you're a physician, please consider making this compassionate adjustment!*

~CHAPTER TWO~

You Have a Choice

MANY PEOPLE, upon being diagnosed, immediately react with fear, and give all their power away to doctors. Contrary to public opinion, the medical establishment, and your own inner doubts, you *do* have a choice about everything: about your doctors, your treatment, your body, what makes you comfortable or uncomfortable. If there were ever a time in your life to claim authority and speak up, this would be it.

Nobody can take your power away unless you allow them to do so. You also have the right to ask the universe for a gentle journey. Set your intention to make it that way, and watch what happens.

This is not always a simple thing to do, especially if you've never considered setting an intention for anything in your life. So, what's the value? By taking the time to be present in the journey on which you're embarking, you get to choose how you want it to go.

The idea is to frame it in a positive way, so that you're moving toward something, i.e., "My intention is for this to be a gentle journey." That's a far better way to phrase it than, "My intention is not to suffer."

It's always wiser to call things into your life in a positive way, rather than capturing them with the word "not." Once again, it's all about the language-ing!

I originally met my surgeon, Terry, in 1997, when I was first told to have my colon removed. There was no pathology, and no one could tell me why it looked so terrible. Initially, I scheduled the surgery, then revisited the decision, and cancelled.

I know I would've survived the surgery but my heart and spirit would've been so broken that I probably would've been dead within a year. Wanting to die — believing that no one could ever love me, that there's nothing to stick around for — is a dark and desolate place to be.

I already knew that most doctors in town wouldn't let anyone else but Terry perform this type of surgery on *them*, so I was comfortable with him. He's not a warm and fuzzy guy. He's extremely direct and perfunctory in his delivery, yet he generously provides a great deal of information and doesn't sugarcoat anything. He is brilliant at what he does, and that was more important than wanting someone to hug.

It had been eight years since that meeting. It was now almost mid-July. Having seen Marilyn, who would become my radiation oncologist, five days earlier, it was becoming clear that surgery was necessary. Quite a shocker, considering I initially had thought that radiation and alternative treatment would be the cure. I was totally blindsided by Marilyn's report.

I don't know if I've ever sobbed like I did that day in her office. The idea of surgery had been so completely off the radar screen for me, and I had to digest all this information as it was being given.

Marilyn set me up with an appointment with Terry. Due to my condition, his examination was extremely painful, and he told me that everything had to go: colon, rectum, and anus. That was more than I had planned to hear.

At one point during the visit, he turned and said, "Let's get you scheduled."

I looked at him and said, "Whoa. This isn't happening before August 15th."

Shocked, he turned to me and said, "Well, I don't know what could possibly be more important than treating your cancer."

I doubt many people ever say no to this man. My eyes welled up, and I looked him in the eye and said, "Spending one last week with my body intact, with the people I love, doing what I love to do. That's more important."

He backed down. Something in him heard me, in the same way that something in me heard him when he told me how he would be failing me as a physician if he made any other recommendation.

"Well," he said, "I guess it won't jump stages in a month."

"I guess not," I replied.

"Well, if you decide to move it up," he added, "You should call."

"That probably won't happen," I said.

My body, at the age of 48, was about to be forever altered. I was certainly not in a huge rush to get cut open.

My advice: don't let anyone bully you into scheduling surgery unless it's a true emergency. Say you need at least a day to think about it. Talk to whomever you need to, in order to process as much as possible about what's going to take place.

Nobody can take your power away unless you allow them to do so.

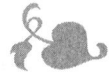

~CHAPTER THREE~

Ask Questions!

FIND SOMEONE you know with a questioning mind, and write down all your questions. Write down everything! If you're able, bring someone with you to every medical appointment, and have them take notes. An objective and detached third party is of tremendous value.

The likelihood of you hearing and remembering everything is greatly diminished when you're the patient. When the time came to tell my sister Patty about the diagnosis, she immediately went into a questioning mode. It was immensely helpful. She was thinking of questions that hadn't occurred to me, and that was wonderful. I ended up making a follow-up appointment with my surgeon, and went in with a written list of questions:

1. What meds will I need? Can I get them in advance—with instructions?
2. What are the meds for?
3. Will they interact well with my thyroid meds? (I've been on those since age 28.)
4. Are there side effects?
5. Will I be going to a local rehab center after my hospital stay?
6. How long might I stay there?
7. What kind of diet will I be on?
8. Will I be able to urinate normally?
9. Will I have to wear special underwear for the anal drainage?
10. Is that something I can get ahead of time, and where?
11. Can a prescription be written so it's covered by my insurance?
12. Will I be able to wear my contact lenses in the hospital?
13. Are you familiar with all the insurance guidelines I might be subjected to?

14. Is your office efficient with insurance paperwork?
15. If the hospital needs to do pre-op stuff with me, who will let them know I'll be out of town before the surgery?
16. When do I get my paperwork for the two-day prep?
17. My primary care physician wanted you to know there is a cyst on my ovaries; does it need to be removed?
18. Do you have positive people whom I can speak to prior to surgery, who have had this procedure?
19. Is the recovery period six to eight weeks from the time of the operation, or does that begin post-op?
20. When will I be able to drive?
21. When will I be able to negotiate stairs?
22. When will I be able to travel?

Terry answered every single question, and my mind was put at ease. Of course, it didn't stop him from saying, "I think you're over thinking this," about halfway through.

Given the fact that my body was about to be permanently altered, I was not quite sure how "over thinking it" could even be possible, but I let it go and continued down my list.

It was another reason to have a list in front of me, so that if I were thrown by any of the answers or potential remarks, I could look down at that piece of paper and know where I left off.

From that point forward, each time I had a doctor's appointment, my sister and I would brainstorm beforehand and come up with questions.

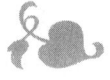

~CHAPTER FOUR~

Securing a Medical Team You Trust

CANCER CAN BE SNEAKY. It doesn't always want to be seen. Before I was first diagnosed, I had been searching nearly three months for an answer to my increasing discomfort. Always willing to embrace alternative methods of healing, I was led to a wonderful woman in Scottsdale. She was a Medical Intuitive, specializing in energetically and psychically reading organs, glands, and blood. There are some very well respected people in this field, and although not embraced by most of the Western medical community, they have a definite place in terms of diagnosis.

She did not see "it" or indicate to me that there was anything serious going on in my lower regions. Three colonoscopies didn't detect "it" either. "It" didn't want to be seen, and I believe there are reasons for that—divine timing being among them.

By December, the pain was so intense that I called Becky, my gastroenterologist, at home, and said she had to see me as soon as possible to do a colonoscopy.

The best thing about great doctors is that they *call you back!* Becky told me to call her office and get on the schedule for the coming week. I was very relieved. Unfortunately, the only thing that showed up was inflammation. Refusing Prednisone (a steroid I consider evil), Becky recommended hydrocortisone enemas to help reduce the inflammation. We planned to speak in a month to see where things stood.

Next to family and friends, your doctors will become the most im-

portant people in your life. Make sure you trust them. Research their backgrounds as you feel necessary for your comfort level.

It was my great fortune that Becky recommended Terry, my surgeon, and Marilyn, my radiation oncologist. Terry and Marilyn decided together that Steve would be the best fit, personality-wise, for me, as an oncologist. Both Marilyn and Steve are part of the same practice, so all my doctors were in communication and on the same page. When they weren't, I made sure to stand up for myself and speak out, so that I was receiving the best care possible.

~CHAPTER FIVE~

Putting Your Affairs in Order— *Before* Surgery

ASK SOMEONE right away to be your team leader, and take that burden off yourself. You need your energy to heal, not to worry about who knows what.

My friend, Kate, actually called me and volunteered to be my team leader. When I asked Kate what that meant she explained that if I provided her with names, phone numbers and e-mail addresses, she would keep those people informed about my surgery and my progress, and help me thank many of them later.

Kate also lent me a walker and a cane, as I was about to have very serious abdominal surgery, which she'd been through with her husband. What a gift! Kate was also able to point me in the right direction regarding whom to call about disability insurance and all the other administrative details requiring immediate attention.

All of this never would have occurred to me.

Providing Kate a contact list also gave me an opportunity to think about the roles that people played, or were going to play, on my medical journey. It was important to have a document listing the names and phone numbers of my friends, my co-workers, and those people taking responsibility for my other affairs, including medical power of attorney (health care proxy), living will and my traditional will. And of course, doctors. All of them.

Make sure you choose well when assigning medical power of attorney. I chose a trio of people, including a friend of mine who is a

nurse, because she would be able to translate any "medical speak," Patty, my sister, because of her questioning mind and our history, and my mom, who absolutely had to be in the room when the doctors were giving information.

❧

IMPORTANT: *Doctors will not give out any information to anyone without a signed medical power of attorney/health care proxy. Saying you are next of kin means nothing without the document.*

❧

Be clear about organ donation. I wrote my wishes on my living will, so that there would be no mistake or assumptions made on my behalf.

After experiencing how long it took to put everything in place, I had to laugh when I thought about how Terry wanted to get me on the table just one short week after the initial diagnosis. What was he thinking — that the medical fairies would come and handle all the insurance, all the disability claims, and getting me a replacement at work?

It ended up taking almost an entire month for everything to be approved and in place. It would have also been a hardship on my family (although they would gladly have done it) to travel from New York to Arizona for such a major event with only a week's notice.

It took me eight years to finally reach the operating table. During that time, my perspective about life shifted and I stopped judging everything as good or bad.

I began asking better questions:

"What is this showing me?"

"Where is the gift in this?"

These questions changed everything for me. And, even though many very experienced healers were indicating that I might not need surgery, I knew, deep down to the core of my being, that the gift *was* the surgery.

~CHAPTER SIX~

Speak Up!

THERE I WAS, post surgery, flat on my back with a colostomy bag, a catheter (fondly termed my pee-bag) and something called a JP bag coming out of me, along with sutures in my vagina from the surgical reconstruction. The irony was not lost on me that after fifteen years of always having to know where bathrooms were located, I now lay in bed without having to find a toilet. I was virtually a walking port-o-potty!

About four weeks following the surgery, my mother and a friend accompanied me on my first visit to Steve, my oncologist. Having never met, he did not know which one of us was the patient. Entering the office, he had the grace to shake hands and introduce himself to my friend, then my mother, then me. I told him my name, and that I was the patient. He then proceeded to spend a full five minutes reading my file as we sat in silence. I thought my mother would have apoplexy.

At one point he said, "Oh. *You're* the lady."

He reached back onto the innumerable stacks of files behind him, grabbed and read two more pieces of paper, and said, "My colleague told me about you. You're very sick."

"Do I look sick?" I replied.

Shocked, he looked at me and said, "No, as a matter of fact, you don't."

"Well, then," I said, refusing to buy into the supposed gravity of the situation.

In his defense, Steve was reading my file, stating my condition as Stage III rectal cancer (out of a possible IV). The hospital staff had told me, "It's as bad a case as we see," and that the doctors were very concerned that it could travel to my liver and lungs.

It was a conscious choice on my part not to go into a tailspin over

that news. I believe that Steve learned a lot that day about treating me as a person, not a piece of paper, and I give him credit for paying attention in a different and better way throughout the entire course of my treatment.

Terry, my surgeon, had told me to ask Steve if I would need a port-o-catheter, which is a device implanted near your left ventricle to guarantee blood flow. Since chemotherapy collapses one's veins, it's a way to avoid a zillion needle sticks that may or may not return sufficient blood for lab work and chemo administration. Steve said yes, and Terry, once again, was to be the attending surgeon.

Terry had said that he wanted to be the determining factor as to when I began treatments. He wanted to ensure that I was healed enough, post-surgery, before I began, because his experience had demonstrated that chemo traditionally slows down the healing process. So I told him I would defer all those decisions to him.

Because my condition turned out to be Stage III, the treatment was going to be very aggressive. Surgery for the port was scheduled for the next Friday. Three days before, Steve's scheduler called and asked if Steve had spoken with me. I said no. She said he wanted me to come in Wednesday, and start my chemo treatments. I told her that the port was being put in on Friday. She said she had told that to Steve, but that he wanted me to start tomorrow.

This is when it's necessary to be fierce. It will serve you well, and it will help them to help you.

I told her to tell him that I was *not* going to come in on Wednesday, that the port was being put in on Friday, and there was no way that I was going to begin treatment without it. I asked her to tell Steve that he could see me any time he wanted to on Monday.

By speaking up, it became *my* decision, and it turned out to be the correct one. I doubt if Terry could have done the surgery during a chemo treatment, which would have lasted three days.

As a result, chemo started the following Monday and was easily administered through my brand new port.

You must speak up. If you're hearing contradictions between doctors, straighten it out right away. Your relationship with your medical

team will greatly improve if you can find it within yourself to properly manage their expectations.

Remember they're human, although it may not always appear that way. Understand how busy they are. It's frightening to realize how many other patients they have.

No matter how much your doctors care about you, there's no way for them to always know what's going on in your file — another reason to stay on top of your own chart and what's happening in your body.

The best ammunition for receiving the best care is when *you* communicate with *them* about your history.

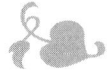

~CHAPTER SEVEN~

Open Your Heart and Call On Your Teachers

WHEN NEWS OF THE PATHOLOGY first came, I called Kimberly, one of my teachers, whom I had known since 1997, the year I was initially told to have my colon removed. She has a background in organic medicine, Jungian psychology, and Native American teachings, and is also a co-founder and Master Teacher of The Way of the Heart.

My voice broke when I said I needed to speak with her about the pathology that just came back. It's a great gift in one's life to have teachers whom you respect and trust. Kimberly had already survived cancer, and had some insight for me about how to proceed.

One of the first things she said was, "You know this isn't your fault." Fortunately, I did know that. I told her about an alternative treatment that Becky had recommended, using frequency, light, and sound vibration. It resonated with us both and I knew I needed to be open to everything that was put in front of me. She also directed me to go into my heart; I had a choice to make about what this was about, and how I was going to travel the path. Great advice, from a great teacher.

Daniel, one of my other teachers, is a true Renaissance man. He has a background in quantum physics, and is gifted in many areas, including music and art. He's the wisest man I have ever known. He said the most profound thing anyone has ever told me: "You know this isn't because you've done anything wrong. In fact, it may very well be because you've done everything right."

Wrap your mind around *that* for a minute.

That one comment completely shifted my perspective, and I invite everyone to consider its truth.

The temptation from the beginning is to ask, "Why me?"

Unfortunately, the only answer to that question is, "Why *not* you?"

We need to ask better questions, which requires reaching beyond the superficial to create a universe that has meaning and embraces all circumstances.

Meaning is everything. Intention, without meaning, is nothing.

When you take the time to assign meaning to whatever you're experiencing, that's when you have the greatest possibility to rise above all that challenges you. When the meaning is more important than the circumstance, you're creating the space for miracles!

What has meaning for you? Why do you want to live? Is it for your kids, your significant other, or a life mission? You need to ask the questions, and you're the only one who can answer them. And, nothing says you have to share this with anyone, even those closest to you. Keep the meaning private, if you so choose. Sometimes, it's gentler to hold things close than to invite in other people's judgment. It's up to you.

It's partly because of Daniel's perspective that I was able to embrace the journey as a gift and a responsibility. What if I were being asked to do this, chosen to do this, simply because I had the strength? What if I were holding this for all those who couldn't?

Suddenly, it felt as though there were truly a higher calling to all of this, and that I could represent the possibility of how to do it well.

So, what does it mean to go into your heart? For me, it was life or death, and very much about choice. Something in me had to really examine what it meant to choose to move forward with love. I had to explore the question more deeply.

What does it mean to me to really love? It's being connected to, and present in my life, and having a desire to live. Or, I could be the drama queen of the century: angry, dark, and a total victim.

The answer to that was a resounding, "No."

It's a downward spiral, and there's no way to heal from that place. Ultimately, as I had a dialogue with my heart, I had the insight that this was *not* about cancer and being sick. It was merely a vehicle to get me to my life mission.

~CHAPTER EIGHT~

Preparing Yourself to Be Unprepared

MANAGING EXPECTATIONS is one of the more challenging aspects of this journey. I prefer the truth in times of great stress. It's easier for me to hear a worst-case scenario than a sugarcoated version, so I can choose the way in which I'd like to manage it.

Treatment is an interesting adventure. Almost immediately, I began to notice things showing up on my body. First, there were mouth sores. Hmmmm. Not so much fun. I wasn't giving them a lot of energy, because I didn't want them to stay around. I used a lot of Listerine. They only lasted a few weeks and went away. My nose. There were times I thought there was a party going on up there that I was simply not invited to! Granted, I live in the desert, and it's dry, but never in my life have I had some form of nose bleed every single day. My radiation oncologist suggested a humidifier, which seemed to help a little. I assume the longer I'm away from treatment, the more it will heal, and ultimately return to normal.

I can't forget mentioning those fried thighs. Nobody tells you this stuff. Not only were they literally blackened from the radiation, but they hurt to the point where I couldn't walk or sit without pain. I used a lot of ointment when I was home, but that's not where I spent most of my day. Ouch!

One day, I couldn't sit at work one minute longer. I called my oncologist's office and told them I must have missed the memo explaining how the pain from radiation escalates about two weeks after treatment ends.

Marilyn examined me and said the skin looked beautiful, but that

I should stay horizontal for a couple of days in order to heal. I took lots of Vicodin during those two days, as the pain was unbelievable.

Advice for your sanity: Although you might desperately need your doctor during an episode like mine, don't call your doctor every time something appears! You'll never get off the phone, and your entire focus will stay on what's wrong, rather than focusing your energy on what's going well. In almost every case, whatever shows up will disappear in a reasonable amount of time.

My approach was to speak with the "invaders."

"Who are you? I've never seen YOU before!"

Things showed up on my face, my arms, and my legs—not all at once, mind you, but almost weekly.

Having a sense of humor about it really helps. It's like having visitors—you're wise to welcome them and be nice, but in the back of your mind, you know they're going to leave!

I was initially told that radiation treatments would be five days a week for five weeks. I mentally prepared myself for that. Ultimately, it was always supposed to be a six-week period (although nobody had said that), and no one bothered to inform me that there would probably be at least a week break about halfway through because one's skin tends to break down and needs some time to heal.

It wasn't a tragedy, but it definitely affected me. I might've prepared myself differently, had I known that everything would be dragged out further than I had planned.

Finally realizing I had to let go of a definite end date to the treatments—that it was out of my control—became a gift. I learned to flow with the challenge rather than raging against it. But I still spoke up when my treatment seemed altered, which happened more than once.

Not long after the incident with my fried thighs, I saw Marilyn again

and told her I wished to be unconscious for the procedure of breaking up of the scar tissue in my vagina. I said I wanted to be sedated, because I knew it was going to be too painful to bear. A couple of weeks earlier, when Marilyn used a tiny dilator to get the right position for the CT scan, I almost came off the table in pain. I couldn't face that again.

Marilyn wanted me to trust her, which I did, and she said that we could work up to it slowly. She scheduled my follow-up before I would see Terry, reminding me that her fingers are smaller for the digital exam. When I asked if there was anything I could do, she said to start with my own finger, but I knew I just couldn't do that. They would have to put me out.

"Marilyn, I'm telling you that I can't do this, and you've never heard those words come out of my mouth." My eyes began to tear up.

She got it. She said she would have to speak to Terry.

"Tell him I'm begging."

"You don't have to beg," she said, as she came over and hugged me.

~CHAPTER NINE~

Welcoming Divine Intervention

I AM NOT, by nature, a religious person. I moved away from organized religion in my early twenties in favor of a spirituality that was neither structured nor bound by institutional limitations. I've always been interested in process, mostly about becoming the best person I am able to be. Opening my heart and mind to this whole journey has enabled me to see the Divine hand in all of it.

The day I was released from the hospital, I was transported by ambulance to a friend's house, where I thought I would be for the four to six week recovery period. The plan called for my mom to join me when my father returned to New York a week later.

When we arrived at my friend's house, I had doubts about whether it was going to be the right place for me to heal. Unfortunately, we had no Plan B, so I knew I was at least spending the night.

My friend is a nurse, and one of the sweetest souls on the planet, so I was confident that if I needed something, I would be in good hands. It was a difficult night, without much sleep for me.

At 6 A.M., I arose, with her help, and had a little piece of bread and some Gatorade. A healthy appetite was not high on my priority list, but I had been told to make every effort, so I did.

About a half hour later, I was in bed and suddenly felt extremely nauseated. I called to my friend, who had the unfortunate experience of entering the room as I vomited up green bile. I was mortified. She got me out of bed to change the sheets and clean up, and brought me into her bathroom, where I took a shower. She stayed with me the whole time, and when I got back into bed, she brought me a bowl, as the nausea was still present.

It didn't take long before the vomiting began again. This was clear-

ly not a good sign, especially since my abdomen was literally stapled together. My friend called my surgeon's office, because I had a feeling that I needed to get back to the hospital.

At first, the woman to whom my friend was speaking said this was probably a one-time thing and suggested that I be given 10 cc's of water every fifteen minutes.

No luck. I was still vomiting, and it was still green bile. On the next phone call, my friend was concerned enough to suggest that we go back to the hospital.

This was part of the exchange:

Woman: "Give her a suppository."

My friend: "Ma'am, she doesn't have a rectum."

Well, that was about it for me. In the midst of all the vomiting and trepidation about the vomiting, a moment of hilarity was presented. This is when you know God has a sense of humor. Needless to say, we called an ambulance and I went back to the hospital.

To this day, I believe that it was the Spirit's way of getting me out of a situation that would not have been conducive to my recovery. It gave me (or, more appropriately, my family) time and space to find a better alternative.

My friend was amazing; I just was not meant to be at her house, which was on the other side of town, a long way from my doctors and most of my friends. It all ended perfectly.

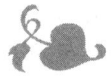

~CHAPTER TEN~

Getting Your Life Back One Day at a Time

THE ONLY WAY to get your life back is to *do* your life!

Terry had said it would be a six to eight week recovery period after the August 18th surgery. Just to be safe, I told my boss that my return date would be November 1st. That left me a little extra margin, in case I was not feeling up to the task.

Having great insurance certainly helped; my caseworker made it very clear that long-term disability would be approved for the extra time past the short-term disability allotment of ten weeks.

The surgery was of greater magnitude than expected, as no one knew that the cancer had breached the vaginal wall. In fact, that was not discovered until five hours into the surgery.

Afterwards, I could do *nothing* by myself. Fortunately, my parents had come out west from New York City. I was instructed to walk every day, and, in addition to my daily shower, I was supposed to take baths to help the drainage wound remain clean.

All of my contraptions made it hilarious, with the pee bag and the JP bag and not being able to freely move with any of it. Sometimes, we just don't know what we're able to accomplish! Without my mother physically in the bathroom with me, I could not have even stepped into the shower. She kept everything in the apartment sterile, running at least four loads (mostly towels) of laundry a day.

Recovery was insane, and that was *before* treatment began.

Each day brought subtle improvements, like walking a little farther or moving better from lying down to sitting up. I was doing pretty well and that was surprising.

My voice had been strong since being in the hospital, which was reassuring to a lot of people I spoke with on the phone who could not be with me in person.

Perhaps, most interesting of all, was noticing the difference between energy and stamina. In the recovery months, it felt as though my physical energy was coming back and doing great.

Ask me to write out checks to pay bills, however, and after about twenty minutes, I had to go lie down and take a nap. It was wild — my brain seemed to be the last part of me to return!

Everyone around me was concerned that I was returning to work too early. But I knew it was the right course of action. Sitting at home and thinking about "it" was serving nothing.

I didn't have the energy to read, so television was my main form of entertainment.

On November 1st, I went back to the office for the first time since before the surgery.

Having had a chemo treatment the day before, I was wearing my chemo pump in its fanny pack around my neck. What a feeling! It was my longest drive to date, and it was my first attempt at climbing thirty stairs. I arrived in time for the 8 A.M. meeting, and my boss introduced me to the woman who had replaced me while I was out, who showed me what I'd missed.

It was wise to only work part-time those first couple of days. My brain was truly the last component to come back into working condition.

Great physical energy but no mental stamina.

It was a lesson in being gentle with myself, and knowing that with time, my brainpower would return.

Another aspect of getting your life back is saying farewell to treatment. Sounds as though it would be an easy task, but it wasn't, at least for me. I'll never forget the incredible kindness that I was always shown from everyone in both Marilyn and Steve's offices.

It was finally time to say goodbye to my chemo pump, which I

wore for two and a half days each treatment, and five days a week during radiation. It was quite the relationship; I couldn't get it wet, so that meant no showers when we were together. It was on me all the time during radiation, either around my neck or by my side, 24/7.

On the day we broke up, I told it I would not be sleeping with it anymore. Wanted to say a proper goodbye, and thank it for all that it had done. Lord knows, I spent more time in bed with that pump than with anything (or anyone) else in the past year!

Closure is important. Take the time to consider all that you have experienced. Breathe it in. Sometimes, doing a form of ceremony can help. For me, it was spending an evening simply saying goodbye to it all, and being grateful for what was ahead. The gifts had far outweighed the negatives. I chose to look at the gifts.

The transition from months of going to treatment, to not going at all can bring up some unexpected issues, as a routine is being broken. Suddenly, you have to redefine what you'll be doing with that time, and how you're going to make it count. You may want to avail yourself of the many resources out there, i.e., support groups or individual counseling. You may feel depressed and lost, especially if you find that the routine ended up defining that time of your life.

Know this: You are not the disease, and there is life after treatment!

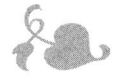

~CHAPTER ELEVEN~

Whose Vagina
Is This Anyway?

AS MY LIFE began to make sense again, I wondered if my sexual life would ever return to normal.

Not long after I returned to work, I was having a conversation with my sister. I was trying to explain how it felt, physically. My bladder was behaving differently, I could still feel the sutures in my vagina, it didn't feel the same, and I was afraid to look. We were both laughing, and I just said it:

"Whose vagina is this, anyway?"

Oh, to have a sense of humor!

Seriously, sexual issues are not something to ignore. If you're the least bit in touch with your sexuality, you'll have questions, and that's okay.

Give yourself permission not to be ashamed!

Personally, I've had to rethink many ideas around sex. I am single, and now wear a colostomy bag. That's a big and permanent change. Unlike most, mine is a permanent ileostomy, with no chance of an inner pouch, as they removed my entire large intestine. Any inner procedure would require more of a regimented eating and irrigation schedule than I am willing to accept. Lord knows, there have been plenty of changes and adjustments, without having to alter my eating schedule. Once again, it goes to personal choice. If you have the opportunity to ask questions about pouch options and what is possible, it may be something you'll wish to consider.

But back to sex.

My vagina was reconstructed in a way that made it smaller. There was no preparation for that, as the breach of the vaginal wall was discovered in surgery, which is when the reconstruction was performed.

There's a possibility of having to break up scar tissue and stretch things

out. My doctors have recommended a few ideas to help with this. It will most likely never be what it once was. That, in turn, is requiring some introspection about the kind of man I wish to attract into my life.

For those of you who are married or in a relationship, it may alter the way in which you engage in sexual activity. It may require counseling, or it may simply be an opportunity to be creative and have fun exploring new ways of giving and receiving pleasure. Perhaps, it will be both. Either way, it's not an area of one's life that should be disregarded.

Would I ever again be able to have sexual intercourse?

For anyone dealing with a cancer diagnosis in the lower body, be it cervical, rectal, vaginal etc., these are serious issues. Not only did the radiation throw me immediately into post-menopause, vaginal reconstruction was still a wild card.

Personally, the thought of being unable to have sexual intercourse would be great cause for grief—not insurmountable, but reason to do some inner work. My hope was that I would not have to grieve, for although things might be different, possibilities still remained.

During a recent visit with my surgeon, I had explained to him that he and Marilyn appeared to be on different pages about this. Terry was saying it would be a tight fit but Marilyn was pointing out that my vagina had been shortened to the extent that I might never be able to have comfortable intercourse again.

When I repeated this to Terry, he said, "That may be true."

"Well, I'm a very sexual being," I replied, "and if that's the case, I need to know so that I can do my work around that."

Terry's conversation in the pre-op area clearly indicated to me that we had different intentions for the procedure. According to him, this was an exam, and if he saw anything that didn't look right, he would be taking biopsies. I was a little stunned, as my intention was for him to break up any scar tissue and to tell me what my options were regarding sexual activity.

When I woke up in the recovery room, my friend told me that everything looked wonderful and there was nothing to biopsy. I was thrilled. At the same time, I didn't feel that I knew anything more than I did going in. My questions remained unanswered.

Soon after, I called Terry's office to make an appointment. Bless his heart, he called me back and took the time to explain what he felt were my options. It's an odd thing to discuss sexuality in a purely clinical manner; however, it was a necessary conversation.

I absolutely understood that if this hadn't been so important to me, Terry probably would have left it at "Everything looked wonderful." But knowing me as he does, he addressed everything. There had been some webbing, but once he broke through that, he could see clear up to the cervix, and everything looked fabulous. The vaginal wall had healed perfectly, and there was no trace of anything that required a biopsy. On the outside, things had healed so well that I looked completely normal.

Regarding sexual function, there was still elasticity, which had been a big unknown. Terry didn't feel that I would have to dilate, as Marilyn had suggested might be necessary, nor did he feel that the scar tissue would grow back.

He went on to say that indeed, I had been anatomically altered, and that common sense should dictate the reality. If it hurt too much, don't do it. He said I may have to explain that to someone. He was concerned with not crossing any professional lines in this discussion, but managed to indicate that some form of practice would help me to know any limitations.

My interpretation? It would be wise to experiment so that I would find out what I needed to know. I love Terry for his willingness to address these things, in spite of the fact that it may have been uncomfortable for him. He was superb.

I felt as though my life had been returned to me. I was healthy, along with the possibility of sexual function. What a gift! It was huge, and glorious, and cause for deep and abiding gratitude.

A new set of circumstances would be forcing me to look at men in a different way. Certainly, there was going to have to be a great

deal more trust before I would be willing to get naked with anyone. Certainly, whoever he might be, he's going to have to show me that he loves me more than he loves what I look like.

This is all new for me, but I'm already seeing the gift in having to have a different set of criteria for having a man in my life.

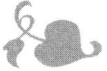

CHAPTER TWELVE

Honoring and Redefining Friendships

FRIENDSHIP has always been one of the most important aspects of my life. Friendship is a sacred trust, one that's not to be taken lightly. People have always trusted me and come to me for advice and/or guidance. Being a "people" person, I always considered that an honor.

During recovery, as I lay in bed, barely able to move, people would call me to check in.

One day, a dear friend was helping my parents get out and shop, as they no longer drive. Mom came back one day and told me that this friend of mine had been diagnosed with diabetes.

My friend had never mentioned anything to me during our phone conversations. I called her immediately and asked why she hadn't told me. She said that she didn't want to burden me, as I had enough on my plate.

I told her, "Honey, I'm lying here with bags coming out of me, barely able to move. Trust me, I have nothing better to do with my time than to be your friend!"

Frankly, I welcomed the opportunity to be of service to someone else, rather than have all the focus on me. It was great to be the helpful one for a change.

Another aspect of the journey was revisiting my ideas around friendship, and who really counted in my life as friends. The most astounding things were happening on a continual basis. People were sending cards and gifts—people I didn't know, hadn't met, or barely had any

contact with. There were the cards from people at work, many who I thought didn't know me very well. Yet, the prayers and good wishes were flowing toward me every day.

I received a card from a friend's sister whom I'd never met, but who felt as though she had known me for the 25-plus years I had been in her sister's life. I cried. It was incredibly moving to receive this outpouring of love.

Somebody described it to me as, "like being eulogized while you're alive."

This was true. I had no idea how loved I was in this world... no idea.

My teacher Daniel put it this way: "Oh, to be broken open to love."

That was what it felt like, and I had never experienced anything like it. The realization struck me that the love is everywhere for everyone, all the time; it's just that most people aren't looking for it, so they don't think it exists. It does, and once you know it, you will see it all the time!

I am at peace. There's a gift in being able to prepare for the end, to decide how to get things in order, no matter what it might be. You have to go for the gifts, for therein lies the salvation, even, and especially, if you know you're terminal.

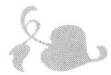

Elizabeth's Love

(Gratitude, Beauty and the Higher Story)

ELIZABETH was in remission until March 2007, when new symptoms emerged. On April 13th, she had surgery to remove a blockage in her small intestine, followed by chemotherapy treatments in May. In early June, Elizabeth was hospitalized for ten days. After a short stay at home, she was re-admitted on June 30th.

On July 10th, one of the attending hospital physicians sat down beside Elizabeth and asked if she had a living will and if she had thought about Hospice. The most recent X-rays had shown no change, meaning her condition could deteriorate rapidly.

The doctor, who had only met Elizabeth twice, looked at her and said, "I think you have one to six weeks."

No one said anything at first.

"It's time to go," said Elizabeth. "This is just no way to live. To do two more treatments and be bald and die anyway—why? This is not living. At least I'll die with hair."

We could only listen.

"There is a readiness. There is still laughter, and joy, and the love will NEVER go away. I'll be in everyone's heart. I don't feel like I'm a coward, it's just time. It's about the truth. It's always been about the truth with me."

While the truth seemed more than her family could bear, Elizabeth faced it straight on. The doctor asked her if there was a person of faith she might want to talk to.

Elizabeth asked the doctor to contact Kimberly and explain the diagnosis.

"I'm not angry about this, thanks to all the love I've been shown in my last two years on earth. Ten years ago I would have been the

angriest little girl. I thank God for what The Way of the Heart has shown me."

Elizabeth asked Kimberly if she would perform a ceremony, which she agreed to do early the following week. The doctor left Elizabeth, our mother and me alone.

"I love you, Mom. You have been the greatest mom ever. I am ready. I am not going anywhere; it's just my physical body. 'Cause I can't do this anymore. I need to be free. It's all good."

From the moment Elizabeth was first diagnosed back in 2005 to what seemed like this final defining moment, she had never reacted in a "poor me, why me" fashion. Instead, she became an inspiration, an oracle, and a sage. Her perspective, words of wisdom and incredible strength humbled us all!

Later that afternoon, while speaking with a friend on the phone from the hospital, Elizabeth said, "Be aware of the gift of time."

Just a few months before, on April 2nd, Elizabeth had celebrated her 50th birthday with family and friends.

"I felt great on my birthday. I felt great the entire weekend. At the party, I was smiling all night long. I felt beautiful and I felt loved. Everything was purple and fabulous! Fifty years old doesn't seem young to me. I've had a full life. Based on the love that's been in my life, it's been a resounding success."

Elizabeth continued calling her friends.

"I am making these calls for completion. I want people to have a choice and not to get a phone call saying that I am gone."

Her words were so profound.

"How can I be sad? To end beautifully... I feel totally complete. I am looking at my life and feeling no regrets. I am being called and my future is on the other side."

Her perspective was amazing.

"I am not afraid. It's going to be beautiful. It's going to be AMAZ-ING, and then I can bring it back to the people who need me. My soul knows it's time. My heart knows I am close. I have no regrets in my life and that's a great thing to say at fifty. I do not feel unfinished about anything. I can accomplish more out of this body, which is failing me."

On July 16th, there was an intimate gathering of family and friends in the chapel of the hospital. Kimberly and Eduardo led the ceremony celebrating Elizabeth's life.

A silver bowl with multicolored pieces of ribbon was passed amongst those who gathered and each person was asked to take a ribbon. Kimberly then asked each of us, one by one, to stand next to Elizabeth and tell her what she had meant to us. After sharing their thoughts with Elizabeth, each person tied their piece of ribbon to the next speaker's. When we were finished, Kimberly placed the necklace of tied ribbons around Elizabeth's neck.

"I came in with love and I'm going out with love. There has been nothing but love for me and the love will go on. It's not about dying. I've never been afraid of dying. I'm at peace with that.

"It's not about being over. It's about the work on the other side. It's all about letting this go and going on to something better. There's beauty in being able to die well, in my way. It's a gift to be able to die in a beautiful and graceful way."

Elizabeth was told to wear this necklace of love for the duration of her life. Kimberly then asked Elizabeth to tell everyone what her life had meant to her. Elizabeth had met with Kimberly and Eduardo the day before the ceremony and had written some notes. She didn't read them at the gathering, but here is most of what she shared with us that day.

"The call of the future is much stronger than the call of the past, and the call to the other side is the future. To have so many people

say to me 'you've been such a model for so many things to me' is amazing.

"Love is everything, yet adversity is the greatest teacher — so, love adversity and know there are always gifts.

"The opportunity for me to see the depths to which I am loved in this world continues to astound me. My family has stepped forward with tremendous courage, respect and profound generosity. My teachers and spiritual family have opened my heart and always call me to a higher and deeper self and story. Gratitude does not adequately describe how I feel about what you mean to me.

"And to my friends and the amazing friendships I have with all of you: thank you for being my compass throughout the years and for allowing me to be who I am.

"I have been blessed to enjoy the beauty and cultures of many places in the world. All of it makes me grateful to live in America, where I have the freedom of choice."

Elizabeth went into inpatient hospice care the next day. Luckily for the people close to her, she stayed with us much longer than the doctor thought. Seven weeks later, on September 5, 2007, Elizabeth was gone.

From the time Elizabeth was diagnosed, through surgery and treatments and remission, when her sickness returned so aggressively until she closed her eyes for the last time, she repeated her mantra again and again.

"It's not about cancer, it's about my life mission."

What was her life mission? To teach people living with illness to find beauty, grace and love; to find the gifts in the time they had left and not to be bitter or angry, but to keep going to the love.

"If that is the gift I can give everyone — to stand up for them-

selves—then that's wonderful. You'll hear my voice telling you to stand up for yourself."

When a friend asked Elizabeth if there was anything she would want to say before she transitioned into the next life—a profound message we could carry with us in our life's journey—Elizabeth, without missing a beat, responded joyfully.

"Run to the Roar."

Her friend asked her what she meant.

"Face your fears. Face your fears or they will kill you."

"And when I'm sad?" I asked her.

"When you feel sad, don't use my name. Save that for when you can say it in a happy moment. The grief you feel is because of the love. Always go to the love."

~Patty Bayer Troup
New York City

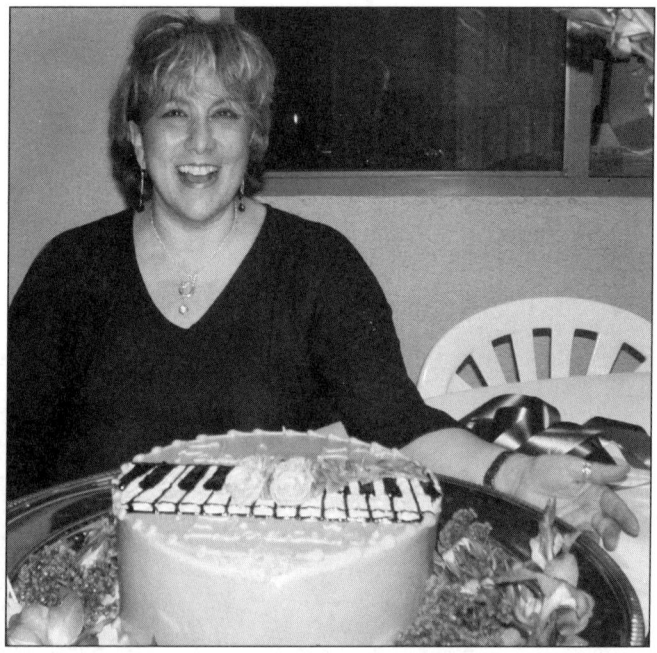

Elizabeth on her 50th birthday

About the Authors

ELIZABETH BAYER was born and raised on the North Shore of Long Island. She graduated from New York University's Tisch School of the Arts in 1979 with a Bachelor of Fine Arts in Theatre. She co-founded *Theco...A Theatre Company* in New York City. While singing pop music in various metropolitan area cabaret venues, Elizabeth was commissioned by the New Theatre of Brooklyn to perform a one-woman show. For many years, she augmented her theatre and songwriting career with work in the advertising and banking worlds.

Elizabeth was introduced to Tucson, Arizona while spending family vacations at a local spa. She eventually moved there in 1991 to begin a new life.

She started working with the Victim Witness program (crisis intervention) in Tucson and remained with them on a volunteer basis for the next eight years. Elizabeth obtained her real estate license in 1993 and published a series of articles in a regional real estate publication.

Elizabeth was designated a Microsoft Certified Systems Engineer from the University of Phoenix in 2000. She was employed full-time as an Executive Assistant for Raytheon.

Elizabeth served as the Southwest Area Coordinator for The Way of the Heart since 2003.

DAVID TABATSKY is a co-author of *Chicken Soup for the Soul: The Cancer Book*. He served as Consulting Editor for *The New York Times* bestseller, *The Right Words at the Right Time: Volume 2, Your Turn*, 101 essays collected by Marlo Thomas. He has written for *The Forward, Par-*

enting, and *Sesame Street Parent* and published two editions of *What's Cool Berlin*, a comic travel guide to Germany's capital.

David teaches theatre at Adelphi University and in New York City public school special education programs.

He lives in New York City with his children, Max and Stella.

Acknowledgments

OUR SINCERE THANKS to Amy Newmark, publisher of Chicken Soup for the Soul, who conceived of including this memoir in Chicken Soup for the Soul's cancer book,

ELIZABETH'S FRIEND, Bruce Kluger, for his professional expertise as a writer and graphic artist,

ELIZABETH'S PARENTS, Eileen and Abba Bayer, for their unbelievable strength, fortitude, nurturing and love,

KENT TROUP for his limitless support, compassion, love and devotion,

And, to all those people who touched Elizabeth's life, we thank you.

~Patty Bayer Troup and David Tabatsky

"Throughout the entire process of treating Elizabeth she was a breath of fresh air for everyone in our office. Elizabeth simply refused to allow massive surgery and aggressive treatments to slow her down. She gave positive meaning to every aspect of her ordeal and her unique perspective benefited us all. I would recommend this book to anyone who has a cancer diagnosis touching their lives."

~Steven J. Ketchel M.D. FACP
Arizona Oncology Associates

www.chickensoup.com